PERIPHERAL DISEASE RECOVERY GUIDE

A Standard Guide On Everything You Must Know From Symptoms, Causes, And How To Treat, Manage, Prevent And More

DR. AIDAN CURLY

Table of Contents

CHAPTER ONE 4

   Peripheral Arterial Disease 4

   What Sort Of Physical Effects Does This Condition Have On Me?..................................12

CHAPTER TWO 17

   What Exactly Causes PAD?............................17

   What Are Some Less Prevalent PAD Causes? 19

   What Variables Put Someone At Risk For PAD?...20

CHAPTER THREE 23

   What Are Some Of The Signs And Symptoms Of PAD?..23

   What About Symptoms Of PAD In Its Advanced Stages? 24

CHAPTER FOUR 27

   What Are Some Of The Risk Factors Associated With PVD?....................................27

   What Are The Possible Side Effects Of PVD? 30

CHAPTER FIVE 33

   Diagnosis...33

CHAPTER SIX	38
How Is PAD Typically Treated?	38
Lifestyle Changes	40
Medications	43
THE END	51

CHAPTER ONE

Peripheral Arterial Disease

Plaque buildup in the arteries in your legs, which carry blood rich in oxygen and nutrients from your heart to your arms and legs, is the cause of peripheral arterial disease (PAD), which is also known as peripheral vascular disease or peripheral artery disease.

Arteries have a smooth inner lining that prevents blood from clotting and promotes consistent blood flow. Arteries are formed in the shape of hollow tubes. When you have peripheral artery disease, plaque (composed of fat, cholesterol, and other substances) slowly forms inside the walls of your arteries, causing them to gradually become more constricted. This plaque can also be referred to as atherosclerosis.

There are numerous plaque deposits that have a tough exterior but a softer interior. Platelets are disc-shaped particles that are found in your blood that help it clot, and they can travel to the area if the hard surface cracks or tears. Your artery could become even more constricted as a result of blood clots that form around the plaque.

If your arteries become constricted or blocked, whether by plaque or a blood clot, blood will be unable to pass through them to nourish your organs and other tissues. This results in damage to the tissues below the blockage, which ultimately leads to their death (a condition known as gangrene). This happens in your toes and feet the vast majority of the time.

The rate at which PAD worsens varies from person to person and is dependent on a wide variety of factors, such as the location in your body where the plaque forms and your general state of health.

What are the factors that increase a person's likelihood of developing peripheral arterial disease?

Tobacco use is by far the most significant risk factor for PAD. In point of fact, people who smoke, either currently or in the past, account for eighty percent of all PAD cases.

When you have one or more of the following risk factors, you put yourself at risk of developing peripheral arterial disease regardless of your gender:

• Regularly using tobacco products (the most potent risk factor).

- Having diabetes.

- Being age 50 and older.

- Having African-American heritage.

- Having a personal or family history of heart disease or a condition that affects the blood vessels.

- Being diagnosed with hypertension (hypertension).

- Having a cholesterol level that's too high (hyperlipidemia).

- Being overweight around the middle.

- Suffering from a problem with how the blood clots.

- Having kidney disease (both a risk factor and a consequence of PAD) (both a risk factor and a consequence of PAD).

Even though peripheral artery disease and coronary artery disease are two separate conditions, they are connected. People who have one are probably also going to have the other. The National Institutes of Health in the United States estimates that a person with PAD has a risk that is six to seven times higher than the average risk for coronary artery disease, a heart attack, a stroke, or a transient ischemic attack (mini-stroke), compared to the average risk for the general population. If a person already has heart disease, they have a one in three chance of also developing peripheral artery disease in their legs.

Not surprisingly, the two diseases also share some risk factors in common with one another. This is due to the fact that these risk factors cause the same changes in the arteries in your arms and legs as they do in the arteries leading to your heart.

As is the case with coronary artery disease, many of these risk factors are beyond your ability to influence. However, according to the findings of the researchers, smoking is the single most important modifiable risk factor for PAD and the complications that can arise from it. Using tobacco products can increase the risk of PAD by 400% and can bring on the onset of PAD symptoms by almost ten years earlier. When compared with non-smokers of the same age, smokers with PAD have a greater risk of passing away from a heart attack or stroke, have a lower chance of survival after undergoing heart bypass surgery procedures on their legs, and are two times more likely to have a limb amputated.

PAD is extremely prevalent, affecting anywhere from 8 million to 12 million people in the United States. Surprisingly, despite the high incidence of PAD, the condition is underdiagnosed and undertreated.

What Sort Of Physical Effects Does This Condition Have On Me?

Claudication is the name given to the typical symptom of peripheral arterial disease (PAD). This is a medical term that refers to pain in your leg that is brought on by walking or exercise and goes away when you rest. Your leg muscles aren't receiving the appropriate amount of oxygen, which is causing the pain.

The dangers posed by PAD go far beyond the inability to walk, and the consequences can be much more severe than missing a shopping trip or a round of golf. The risk of developing a wound on the legs or feet that does not heal when treated increases when a person has peripheral artery disease. In the most severe cases of PAD, these sores can progress into areas of dead tissue, known medically as gangrene, which ultimately makes it necessary to amputate the affected limb (either the foot or the leg).

The effects of PAD can extend beyond the limb that is directly affected due to the interconnected nature of the circulatory system in your body. It is common for people to have atherosclerosis in other parts of their bodies if they have it in their legs. People who have peripheral artery disease have an increased risk of suffering a heart attack, stroke, transient ischemic attack (mini-stroke), or problems with the arteries that supply their kidneys (renal arteries).

People who have PAD have an increased risk of developing serious health problems if they do not receive treatment, including the following:

• A heart attack is permanent damage to the muscle of your heart caused by a lack of blood supply to your heart for a period of time that is prolonged.

• A stroke is when there is a disruption in the blood supply to your brain.

A transient ischemic attack, also referred to as a TIA, is a temporary disruption in the blood supply to your brain.

A narrowing or blockage of the artery that supplies blood to your kidneys, also known as renal artery disease or stenosis.

• Amputation refers to the surgical removal of a portion or all of a person's toes, feet, legs, or arms (the arm is removed surgically only very infrequently), most frequently occurring in people who also have diabetes.

CHAPTER TWO

What Exactly Causes PAD?

The most common reason for peripheral arterial disease (PAD) is a blockage in the arteries, which are the blood vessels that lead away from the heart. This medical condition is known as atherosclerosis. It occurs when substances in your bloodstream, such as fat and cholesterol, form plaques that build up in your arteries and cause blockages.

The majority of plaque is composed of fat, and at first it has a waxy consistency. They amass very gradually, to the point where you are oblivious to their presence. Plaque buildup, which occurs over time, causes your arteries to become stiffer and more narrow. It's very similar to having outdated plumbing in a house. If there is gunk in the pipes, water will drain more slowly, and the pipes will eventually become clogged. When plaque builds up in your arteries, the flow of blood is reduced, and your body does not receive the oxygen it requires.

Plaque doesn't form for a reason that's completely clear to medical professionals. They believe that it is a disease that progresses slowly and that it may have begun in childhood.

What Are Some Less Prevalent PAD Causes?

If you do not have atherosclerosis, your doctor may begin to look for other risk factors, including the following:

• An infection or inflammation of a blood vessel; • An injury to your arms or legs; • An irregular shape of your muscles or ligaments (the tissue that connects your bones or joints together); • Exposure to radiation;

What Variables Put Someone At Risk For PAD?

If you already have heart disease, you have a chance of having PAD that is one in three. The following are some additional risk factors for developing PAD: • Your age (older than 50)

• Diabetes

• High cholesterol

• High blood pressure • Obesity • Lack of physical activity • Smoking • Not being active enough

In what ways does smoking contribute to PAD?

Your smoking habit is the single most important risk factor for PAD that is under your control. When compared with people who don't smoke, your chances of developing PAD are increased by a factor of 400. And in patients who have PAD, smokers are more likely to experience symptoms ten years earlier than nonsmokers do.

In addition, smokers who have PAD fare worse after certain types of heart bypass surgery, are twice as likely to require limb amputations, and have an increased risk of passing away from a stroke or heart attack.

Have a conversation with your primary care physician about the various medications and treatments that can assist you in quitting smoking.

CHAPTER THREE

What Are Some Of The Signs And Symptoms Of PAD?

Because there is less blood flow to your legs, you might experience pain or cramping in your muscles. The term for this kind of discomfort is claudication. It is most noticeable when you are moving, such as when you are walking or climbing stairs; however, it disappears when you stop moving.

It can affect a variety of muscle groups, including the buttocks and hips, calves (the most common site of involvement), feet (less common), and thighs.

What About Symptoms Of PAD In Its Advanced Stages?

Burning or numbness is a sensation that can be experienced by some individuals. If you have an advanced form of PAD, you may experience discomfort in your toes or feet even when you are resting.

Other signs and symptoms may include the following: changes in the color of your legs; erectile dysfunction, which is most common in men with diabetes; leg weakness; fatigue while walking, especially in legs; legs that are cooler than your arms; one leg that feels colder than the other; loss of hair on your legs; a fainter pulse in your feet; shiny skin on your legs; skin that looks pale or kind of blue; slow toenail growth; wounds or sores on your toes or feet that

If you have peripheral arterial disease (PAD) in your arms, you will experience symptoms that are comparable to those in your legs. During physical activity, you might experience discomfort in the form of pain, cramps, or heaviness;

however, these sensations will go away once you stop moving.

You might find that your hands are numb or cold, and that the tips of your fingers look blue or white. In addition to this, you could have wounds on your arms and hands that do not appear to heal.

There are some instances of severe blockages in which the individual feels no pain at all. In most cases, this occurs because your body grows new blood vessels around the obstructions.

CHAPTER FOUR

What Are Some Of The Risk Factors Associated With PVD?

There are a lot of different things that can put you at risk for PVD.

If any of the following apply to you, you have an increased likelihood of developing peripheral vascular disease (PVD): • you are over the age of 50 • you are overweight • you have abnormal cholesterol levels • you have a history of cerebrovascular disease or stroke • you have heart disease • you have diabetes • you have a family history of high cholesterol, high blood pressure, or PVD • you have high blood pressure • you have kidney disease that requires hemodialysis • you have a history of PVD

Some of the behaviors that contribute to an increased risk of developing PVD are as follows: not engaging in physical activity; having poor eating habits; smoking; and using drugs.

Claudication

Claudication is one of the most typical signs of peripheral vascular disease (PVD) and peripheral arterial disease (PAD). Walking can cause pain in the muscles of the lower limbs, which is known as claudication. You might become aware of the pain when you are walking more quickly or for longer distances. After getting some rest, the problem usually disappears. When the pain returns, it might take the same amount of time as before for it to go away.

Claudication is a condition that develops when the muscles that are being used do not receive an adequate supply of blood. When someone has PVD, their blood supply is restricted because their vessels are so narrow. This causes more problems when there is movement involved than when there is no movement involved.

Your symptoms will become more severe and occur more frequently as your PAD condition worsens. After some time, you may even experience pain and fatigue while you are resting. Inquire with your physician about the various treatments that could help improve blood flow and decrease pain.

What Are The Possible Side Effects Of PVD?

The complications that can arise from PVD that has not been diagnosed or treated can be severe and even be fatal. When blood flow is restricted due to PVD, this can be an early warning sign of other forms of vascular disease.

Complications of PVD can include the following: death of tissue, which can result in amputation of a limb; impotence; pale skin; pain at rest and with movement; severe pain that restricts mobility; wounds that don't heal; unhealing wounds; life-threatening infections of the bones and blood stream; wounds that don't heal.

The arteries that supply blood to the brain and heart are the source of the most serious complications that can arise. It is possible for these to become clogged, which can lead to a heart attack, a stroke, or even death.

CHAPTER FIVE

Diagnosis

In order to diagnose peripheral artery disease, your doctor might rely on some of the following tests:

• A physical examination. During a physical exam, your doctor may find signs of PAD, such as a weak or absent pulse below a narrowed area of your artery, whooshing sounds that can be heard over your arteries that can be heard with a stethoscope, evidence of poor wound healing in the area where your blood flow is restricted, and decreased blood pressure in your affected limb. Your doctor may also find evidence of poor wound healing in the area where your blood flow is restricted.

- Ankle-brachial index (ABI) (ABI). The diagnosis of PAD frequently makes use of this particular test. The blood pressure in your arm is compared with the blood pressure in your ankle.

A standard blood pressure cuff and a specialized ultrasound device are both utilized by your doctor in the process of obtaining a reading of your blood pressure and determining blood flow.

To get an accurate picture of how severely your arteries are constricted while walking, you can walk on a treadmill while having readings taken both before and immediately after the exercise.

• Ultrasound. Doppler ultrasound is one type of the specialized ultrasound imaging techniques that can help your doctor evaluate the flow of blood through your blood vessels and identify any arteries that are blocked or narrowed.

• Angiography. During this test, a dye is injected into your blood vessels, and your doctor is then able to observe the flow of blood through your arteries in real time. Using imaging techniques such as X-rays, magnetic resonance angiography (MRA), or computerized tomography angiography, your doctor will be able to track where the dye is traveling in your body.

An invasive procedure called catheter angiography involves injecting dye into the affected area after threading a catheter, which is a thin, hollow tube, through an artery in the groin of the patient. With this particular kind of angiography, your physician will be able to treat a blocked blood vessel at the same time that they diagnose it. Your doctor will first locate the section of the blood vessel that is constricted. Next, he or she will either widen the vessel by inserting a very small balloon and causing it to expand, or by giving you medication that increases blood flow.

• Blood tests. A sample of your blood can be used to diagnose diabetes, determine your cholesterol and triglyceride levels, and measure both of these.

CHAPTER SIX

How Is PAD Typically Treated?

When treating PAD, the primary objectives are to reduce the risk of heart attack and stroke, as well as to improve quality of life by reducing the pain that is associated with walking.

You can prevent PAD from worsening by getting treated, getting an early diagnosis, and making changes to your lifestyle. In point of fact, a number of studies have demonstrated that it is possible to reverse the symptoms of peripheral vascular disease through the combination of physical activity and vigilant management of both cholesterol and blood pressure. Talk to your primary care physician, a vascular medicine specialist, or a cardiologist as soon as possible if you suspect that you may be at risk for peripheral arterial disease (PAD) or that you may already have the disease. This will allow you to begin a program for either prevention or treatment as soon as possible.

Your PAD can be treated with changes to your lifestyle,

medication, and even interventional procedures.

Lifestyle Changes

Making changes to your lifestyle to cut down on your risk factors is an important part of the initial treatment for PAD. Among the many adjustments you can make to better manage your condition is to give up using tobacco products. Talk to your healthcare provider about the different smoking cessation programs that are offered in your area.

• Consume a diet that is both well-balanced and low in cholesterol, fat, and sodium while having a high fiber content. You should not consume more than 30 percent of your total daily calories from fat. A maximum of seven percent of your daily calorie intake ought to come from saturated fat.

Avoid products made with trans fats, including those made with partially hydrogenated and fully hydrogenated vegetable oils. If you are overweight, losing weight will help you lower your overall cholesterol while simultaneously raising your HDL, or "good," cholesterol level. You might need the assistance of a registered dietitian in order to make the appropriate dietary adjustments.

- Exercise. Start a consistent exercise routine, such as going for walks.

The treatment of PAD can be helped by walking, which is an extremely important activity. People who walk frequently should anticipate a definite improvement in the amount of distance they are able to walk before experiencing pain in their legs.

- Take care of any additional medical conditions you have, such as high blood pressure, diabetes, or high cholesterol.

- Try to maintain a low level of stress. Exercising, yoga, and meditation could be helpful in this regard.

- Take proper care of your skin and feet in order to reduce the likelihood of developing complications and avoid infections.

Medications

- Medication that helps lower cholesterol. Statins are cholesterol-lowering medications, and one option for lowering your risk of heart attack and stroke is to take one.

People who suffer from peripheral artery disease should strive to bring their levels of low-density lipoprotein (LDL) cholesterol, also known as "bad" cholesterol, down to less than 100 milligrams per deciliter (mg/dL) or 2.6 millimoles per liter (mmol/L). This is the goal. If you also have other major risk factors for heart attack and stroke, such as diabetes or if you continue to smoke cigarettes, your goal should be even lower.

• Medication for treating high blood pressure If you also have high blood pressure, your doctor may decide to prescribe you blood pressure medication in order to bring it down.

The target range for your blood pressure medication should be lower than 130/80 millimeters of mercury (mm Hg). This is the recommended course of action for those who suffer from coronary artery disease, diabetes, or chronic kidney disease. Achieving a blood pressure reading of 130/80 mm Hg should also be the goal for healthy adults aged 65 and older, as well as healthy adults aged under 65 who have a 10% or higher risk of developing cardiovascular disease within the next 10 years.

- Medication for the regulation of blood sugar If you have diabetes, maintaining control of your blood sugar levels is even more crucial for your health. Have a discussion with your primary care physician about the blood sugar goals you have set for yourself, as well as the steps you need to take in order to reach those goals.

- Medications that prevent the formation of blood clots. It is essential to enhance blood flow to your limbs because peripheral artery disease is linked to a decreased amount of blood flow.

Your physician may recommend a regimen of daily aspirin treatment or another medication, such as clopidogrel (Plavix).

• Medications for the relief of symptoms Cilostazol is a medication that thins the blood and widens the blood vessels, both of which contribute to an increase in the blood flow to the limbs. Patients suffering from peripheral artery disease often find relief from their leg pain after using this medication. This medication is known to occasionally cause side effects such as headaches and diarrhea.

An alternative to cilostazol is pentoxifylline (Pentoxil) (Pentoxil). This medication is not known to cause many adverse effects, but it is not considered to be as effective as cilostazol.

angioplasty, as well as surgery

In certain instances, angioplasty or surgery may be required in order to treat peripheral artery disease, which is the root cause of claudication:

• Angioplasty. During this procedure, a catheter is inserted into a blood vessel so that it can be guided to the affected artery. At this point, a tiny balloon at the tip of the catheter is inflated in order to compress the plaque against the artery wall, reopen the artery, and increase blood flow all while the artery is stretched open.

In addition, your physician may choose to place a mesh tube, also known as a stent, within the artery to assist in maintaining its patency. This is the same method that doctors employ in order to open arteries in the heart.

- Surgical by-passing. A blood vessel from another part of your body or a synthetic vessel might be used by your doctor in order to create a detour around the blocked artery in your body. With the help of this method, the blood can flow around the constricted or blocked artery.

• The use of thrombolytic therapy. If you have a blood clot that is blocking an artery, your doctor may inject a clot-dissolving drug into your artery at the point where the clot is located in order to break up the clot and restore blood flow.

THE END

Printed in Great Britain
by Amazon